What The Physician Whispered

including

The Chief Poisoner Will See You Now

a chapbook of poems

Ron Louie

Seattle, 2025

ISBN # 979-8-9939539-1-5. Publisher: Ron's Nonplussed

Print format

Self-Publisher's Note: The chapbook title is a play on the first poem, "What the Magician Whispered" (which appeared online 2022: *A Closed Eye Open*, https://theclosedeyeopen.com/).

Any typos, formatting issues (damn TOC) , errors, or omissions in the chapbook might just be intentional, "poetic license," or due to the optometrist's latest prescription. The character portrayals are fictions. Except when clearly stated or quoted, no identification with actual persons (except self and family, living or deceased) should be inferred. The other characters and events are basically products of my imagination; any resemblance of characters to real persons (without permission) is purely coincidental. Some previously published poems will look different here because of design constraints, but it's adaptability, right?

Advice to the Reader: the poems are grouped into roughly thematic sections, separated by photos. It might be more palatable to read a section, put the thing down, and pick it up later, but please do pick it up again.

The late poet Robert Wallace taught that many poems are revealing about the poet. He also taught that poems are best when read out loud.

Contents

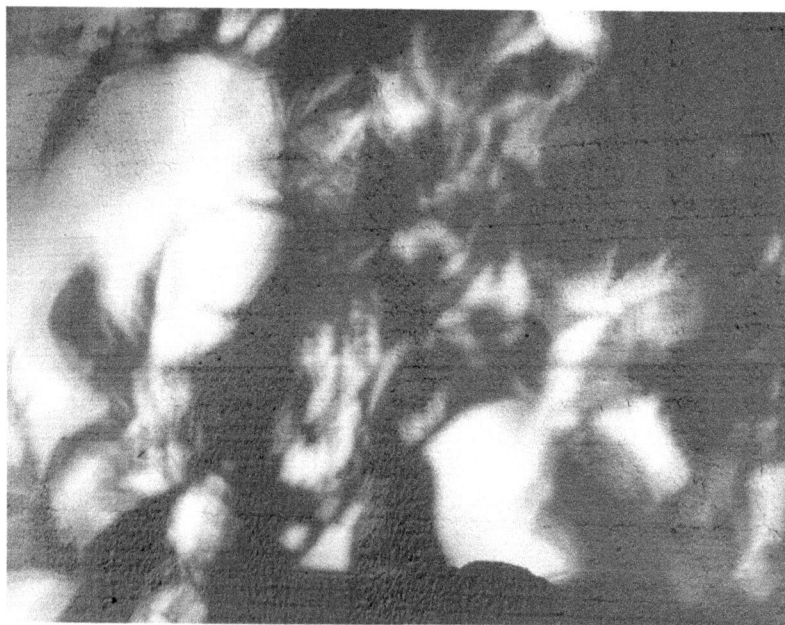

I.

What the Magician Whispered

You may think it's here, or there, but it's not.
I try to make the transpositions zing.
Even before we've met, I'm ahead of you.
But I'm trying to please you. Really.

Productions and vanishes might just be
two sides of a coin; although our eyes
are seemingly made to look forward,
our minds can't help thinking back. Really.

What you think, how you choose,
whether it's conceptual, numerical,
or a value, it will be something I might
just influence with words. Really.

You might not want to be pleased.
If my method is transparent to you,
perhaps you see that I'm striving
to avoid disenchantment. Really.

Tonio: Telling Time

What did he already know, straddling his mother's broad lap, hiding
his face, listening at our halting and stuttering and murmuring babble,
the nonsensical sounds of statistics and "choices" rushing like noise,

perplexing his parents past their own understanding,
shifting from one leg to the other, unfathomed,
watching the waters well up around him, then spill,

Of the future, for the first time foreseen,
far from the red-and-blue striped swingsets
and the ants and the pebbles at the playground,

far from the bright candy wrappers at the deli,
and his mother's silken neck, where he
loved to rub his hot cheek?

Tonio turned, eyes wide, cried and clung a while,
his tears obscuring the flood of our own fears.
Slowly the quietness of the small room returned.

He had spied the box of silly, tattered toys;
he wanted them, right now, endearing just for the present,
silent of their own irrelevant past.

Chief Complaint: He Predicts Earthquakes

Everyone there, except the pediatrician, spoke two or more languages.
For each child, staff would list the medical issue, a terse "chief complaint,"
using the parents' own words, on why they were seeing a Western doctor,
since the children didn't, wouldn't or couldn't complain for themselves.

It's a parent's concern, via a native vernacular, through an interpreter's ear,
twisted with some medical phrasing, a flashing linguistic triple flip,
leaving the doctor to decipher the situation for clinical intervention,
a contorted tumbling run, with the expectation of a two footed landing.

And this one predicted earthquakes. Taller and chubbier than expected,
the child hovered outside the door, apparently shy about entering the room,
already crowded with his mother, an aunt, an interpreter, and a doctor.
He predicted earthquakes often; but his uncanny timing scared people.

He spoke no English, hardly spoke at all, rocking, snuffling and shuffling,
sometimes whining like a wet puppy trying to open its eyes.
His own eyes closed when someone spoke. When they did open,
they didn't seem to see, or maybe they were seeing too much.

Did he really use the word "earthquake," or was it "moving ground" in the
language of his family, or was it more figurative? Did he feel dizzy, did he
hear things, or was he trembling, perhaps having a seizure, or did he just
have tingling in his toes? This lad was "special," we all knew it,
and each one of us already had an interpretation.

How does one diagnose human earthquake prediction, at any level:
as misconstrued, or statistical aberration, or savant-like behavior?
Or explain cultural expectations of conduct, or communication gaps in
children while using different languages, or the deliberate limitations
of a medical mindset, all whilst using fewer syllables?

So we did what we usually do, approach understanding clumsily,
not knowing if such a complaint could ever be resolved, or how,
or to whose satisfaction, or the child's own wishes, with so little help
to offer, recording an uncertain prognosis, so awkward to translate,

entering the clinical elements anyway, using terms that burnish
our bronzed mode of medical thinking, closing our own eyes,
trying to comprehend his vision, or the way his world might move.

Couplets to a Pre-Existing Condition

O Solomon! what wisdom is needed for that physician
who deals with a child and a "pre-existing condition":
of all known miseries, the one that presupposes
a definable beginning, and presumptively imposes
a linear relationship of time
to illness, with no respect for the sublime
that turns lugubrious, ending with antecedents circular,
and predicated upon a bureaucratic vernacular;
Which for the peripatetic pediatrician
presents a peculiar imprecision:
when caring for very sick children or infants,
with cystic fibrosis or leukemia, for instance,
whose spirits hold hostage parental emotions;
are these children just some post-conceived notions,
begging their epistemic question, with exons existential,
full of knowing and pre-knowing, (the code confidential)?
Can we now really judge origins, without pre-maturity,
or assess a person's, or a population's risk-pool purity,
and not mock the politics of self-determination?
Yet Media-tricians trumpet the research's implication
for these progenitor cell products in our age of new genetics;
these innocently assorted alleles, (admittedly, at times pathogenic),
whose critical pre-existing condition is birth,
with no consideration of bottom-line net worth?

Missing Any Thing

for K.I.

That blade of grass, that one, grew, but I missed it.
This tree, beyond embracing, grew wider, but I missed it.
You grew too, I was there, but I missed it.
Now something else is happening,
It seems the opposite of growing, for you.
For me, it's palpable, it's measurable,
it's almost inconceivable, but it's unavoidable;
vainly missing no thing, every thing, any thing.

The Chief Poisoner Will See You Now

You are looking at me, little one,
perhaps wondering who I might be.
Even though I might seem friendly,
you seem wary and frightened, not yet
used to seeing strangers and busy places.
Someone thought maybe I might help save you.

I offer to give you poison.

They have not told you, because they do not know
how sick you really are, meaning how close you are
to an unexpected conclusion that no one wishes for you,
not even me, whose feelings you cannot know.
Someone must trust that I have fortune-telling skill;
maybe they heard I have seen others this sick.

What I have is poison.

Why you are here, why they brought you now,
why you got sick, how it is that my offering is poison,
why sweets or being good or smiles won't work as well,
are all good questions, which I cannot answer.
Who you are, who you will be and what will happen
are all good questions, which I cannot answer.

I do know poison, and can give you details.

I am not saying you must be poisoned here.
Here is where you are. You can go elsewhere.
But someone asked me, and I honestly know of no
better or faster way than poison for the effect
we presume you want, without your saying it.
Poison might do for you; it is not for everyone.

The poison stands ready.

People speak of belief in this circumstance
belief is not required for poison to have effect.
You may not believe me either, or the story I can tell
about how poison might cure, the irony and oxymoron.
It is just a story, serving an irrational need, but
you will ultimately decide its reality or fiction.

We have poison, you or someone tell us when to start.

Poison is not given lightly, one does not take it easily.
As Chief Poisoner, I will be nearby often enough,
but I must tell you, I delegate many tasks,
especially the manipulation of euphemisms.
Words I use might seem harsh, like bitter concoctions,
but are used, of course, for effect.

We have poison, but no promises.

Your circumstance is not unique,
but you, little one, are unique. I am not flattering you;
we respect your specialness, your individuality, and
therefore cannot predict all the effects of poison on you.

We can use chocolate syrup sometimes,
not always, if you really think that might help.

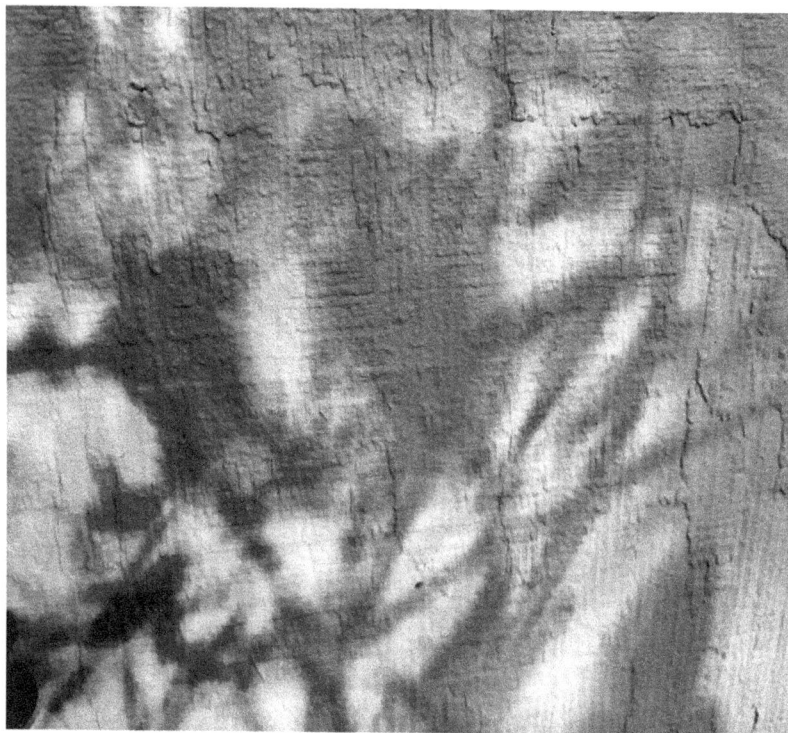

II.

Matter of Fact

Her face was matter of fact when she heard the pronouncement.
The neuropsychologist was her colleague; he remained professional,
but slipped in some sympathy with the data, which I could not appreciate.

She didn't display a mask of depression, or Parkinson disease.
Her face remained pliable, not pleased, but neither terribly pained,
no exhibition of perplexity, or petulance, or surprise, a pensive look,
retaining its complex grace, a quiet reserve, a solemn alertness,
the beauty of humane consciousness, with no further expectations.

In her own practice, she had encountered early Alzheimer disease first
hand: that wonderful younger woman, whose baby she had delivered,
working in accounting until the numbers became exotic, then alien;
she had told me about that patient, with shock, sadness, and resignation.

But I didn't understand this. I wouldn't. It was the guy, his tests, the setting.
At home, I made her try to draw a clock, count backward, recite words, and
copy intersecting rectangles. She tried, this good doctor who had always
bested me in calculus, organic chemistry, and marriage. She wasn't angry.

So how could I be mad? She was setting the example, as she had done
her whole life, her whole career, without pessimism or regret, or fanfare,
just ready to go on, even though her words and steps might mutate,
unpredictably, ever aware of the possible endpoints, with each of us
now grappling this present moment, trying to recognize its identity.

Dedicated to IRJ; suggested by Meryl Comer

Handwashing 03:47

At this time of night, my hands
know what to do, stubbornly,
poorly pre-programmed
but compelled and automatic still,
with the cold bracing water
and the glop of scented soap
unable to break their rhythm,
movements purposeful and synchronized,
not just the deep creases of the palms
but the six webs between the eight fingers
counting the thumbs separately,
each grabbed by the opposing fist
bent with friction and twisted firmly
then sliding each cupped palm
around the flesh beneath the shortest fingers,
surprisingly cooler than anywhere else,
gliding across the dorsal latticeworks,
before moving down to surround each wrist
around and around to a vague spot
they both know, halfway to the elbow,
with an unthinking brushing of fingerpads
and thumbs against ten shorn nails
finally plunging it all
under what is thought to be a glistening absolution,
believing that traces of the past
can be further diminished.
The hands are now ready to be dry again,
ready to go again
no matter what just finished at 03:44.

Alzheimer Retrogenesis as Oxymoron

Reading the term "retrogenesis" aloud caused me a spasm,
an unthinking oscillatory movement, twisting my head
from left to right, just slightly, with a concomitant rotation
upward from my red-rimmed globes within their bony orbits,

and a simultaneous utterance one might describe as dysphoric.
One would not call it a seizure or Tourettistic, exactly, but
how dare those scientists brain us by combining opposing concepts,
going backward while starting anew, so make up your minds people!

But maybe their minds are really made that way,
starting not from zero but from some previous notions,
acknowledging a history, thinking backward before an astounding
action like taking that forward first bite of the apple.

Because Genesis I get, even though, strangely,
the etymology of genesis coincidentally
insinuates the view of a tyrannical
Deoxyribonucleic Acid, dictating to its lackey

transcriptionists and translators all the schemes,
subterfuge, and machinations that it holds so close,
in its own code, presumably written long before
it is awakened to unleash its autocratic power.

And Retro I get, with the salient example of Lot's wife, forever now
a stark crystalline image, looking back to Sodom of all places,
a severe sanctioning for regarding the past, a cognitive choice,
whether precipitated by her own tears or perhaps a glint in her eyes.

But retrogenesis, that portmanteau, for the progressive loss
of abilities, this term for the idea that this devastating deterioration
is the delight of development stuck in a reverse gear,
notably deficient in joy or accomplishment, I don't get.

The Bard had a similar idea, though, centuries ago. Even with current
notions of neuropathophysiology, and therapy, we do not escape a
"second childishness… sans teeth, sans eyes, sans taste, sans everything."

[Reisberg, B., Franssen, E., Hasan, S. et al. (1999). Retrogenesis…brain aging,
Alzheimer's…. Eur Arch Psy Clin Neurosci. DOI: 10.1007/PL00014170]

Status Report to Insurance: Incontinent

She is otherwise OK, eating a bit better, but still not standing.
Sleep is interrupted; last night she was vocalizing at 0100, 0530, 0700;
she seems to sleep quietly in between those times.

Assessing quality of life, one wonders how she might think of her own now,
since she was a doctor who took care of Alzheimer's and other dementias.
Now she needs hand feeding, with the application of gentle pressure,

just to get the stamp-sized apple, or shredded chicken, or chewy chocolate
into her inattentive mouth, eyes open, but gazing elsewhere, never at food,
bobbing her head. If she accepts it and starts chewing, one might ask her

if it tastes good; one may observe an audible "mmm" and raised eyebrows.
When she refuses food, with pursed lips, one concedes to the complexity
of perceptions and physiology and the dueling agendas of the moment.

She even smiles sometimes, says "hi" and nods in seeming recognition
sometimes, but sometimes seems irritated or angry, when her vocalizations
have volume, tonality, and fluidity, a vocabulary of unfamiliar syllables;

she is perhaps quieter than the level documented six months ago.
Her daily rhythms and tardive repetitive movements are all about the same,
on fewer meds; the others didn't help or seemed to make things worse.

It's Not Now Fashionable To Regret What I Didn't Say

By now I haven't said what others might have said
to you
but they said it to others, not you
or maybe they wrote it, and said it better of course,
what I wouldn't say, not
that I couldn't say.

But now I remember everything you never said
to me
that I thought I wanted to hear you say, because
you would never write it, but no one could ever say it
better, at least for me, I realize that now,
even if I wouldn't hear it then.

And now I barely remember anything I did say
to you
as when we tried to peer through the jagged dingy window
of that old house we both admired so much
or tried to squint through the lace-like cracked glass
of your smashed parked car, rammed by some idiot.

For now I know that when you wouldn't even look
at me
no one could say there would be this present perspective,
embracing us both, of who we were for each other, or would be,
since here you are, and I am here,
but we can no longer talk, or even listen, the way we could.

Counting to Himself, Again

In the non-erotic intimacy of that moment,
undressing her, drying her, enduring the wait,
he was naturally counting to himself, again.

He knew that it was a device for distraction,
mentally counting in reverse, with un-numbered
missteps and restarts, fleeting the seconds away,

that serial subtracting by threes or sevens
was not a practical skill, but testing, some earnest
attempt to calculate a person's conditional status,

even after the journey had already begun down that slide,
not fast enough for fun, or terror, the ride imperceptible,
yet so futile trying to claw a way back up.

Knowing someone is sliding cannot halt the slippage.
Counting down is not retrospection, it's just something to do,
as artless as typing away at transience non-metrical.

For the duo in the non-erotic intimacy of that moment,
one of them is counting again; perhaps now both are,
driven by some shared subconscious pulse.

Caregiving: Dancing vs. Wrestling Moves

It looks like a "staggered stance lift," if a referee were
to score us, although I'm trying my best to be gentle,
picking her up from a deep chair, her eyes half-closed.

Maybe the scorekeeper thinks I've asked her to dance.

After all, we have music playing, and as the lift proceeds,
I'm counting out loud, "one and two and three and…"
Her legs don't quite buckle, and I can feel that she's trying.

She used to smile, like a reflex, when she could dance,
sometimes swaying just by herself, some inner music
to which I never had access, so it's not that different now.

Maybe she is smiling; I just can't see because I'm holding her
up too close, my arms flexed like biceps curls, under her arms.
It's sometimes wet after her face rests against my shirt.

I don't look down to see if she's moving her feet, but
rely on the sensation they are not dragging. I'm concentrating
on my own balance, trying to prevent a non-scoring fall.

A musical syncopation pertains, as we cut across the carpet
to the couch, prepared with three pads, the bottom wet-proof,
and three pillows. The move is to turn her, then lay her down.

Maybe the official thinks we are about to score points.

Ancient wrestlers were legendary: the Bible had Jacob,
wrestling his Angel all night; Heracles grappled Death.
Goddess Palaistra championed our art and skill.

We are not now being Biblical, or Olympic, or even competing,
but the daily sequences, the maneuvers, and the holds
all get the intimate job done; we clinch the end of the round.

Maybe the timekeeper neglects the bell, so the music plays on.

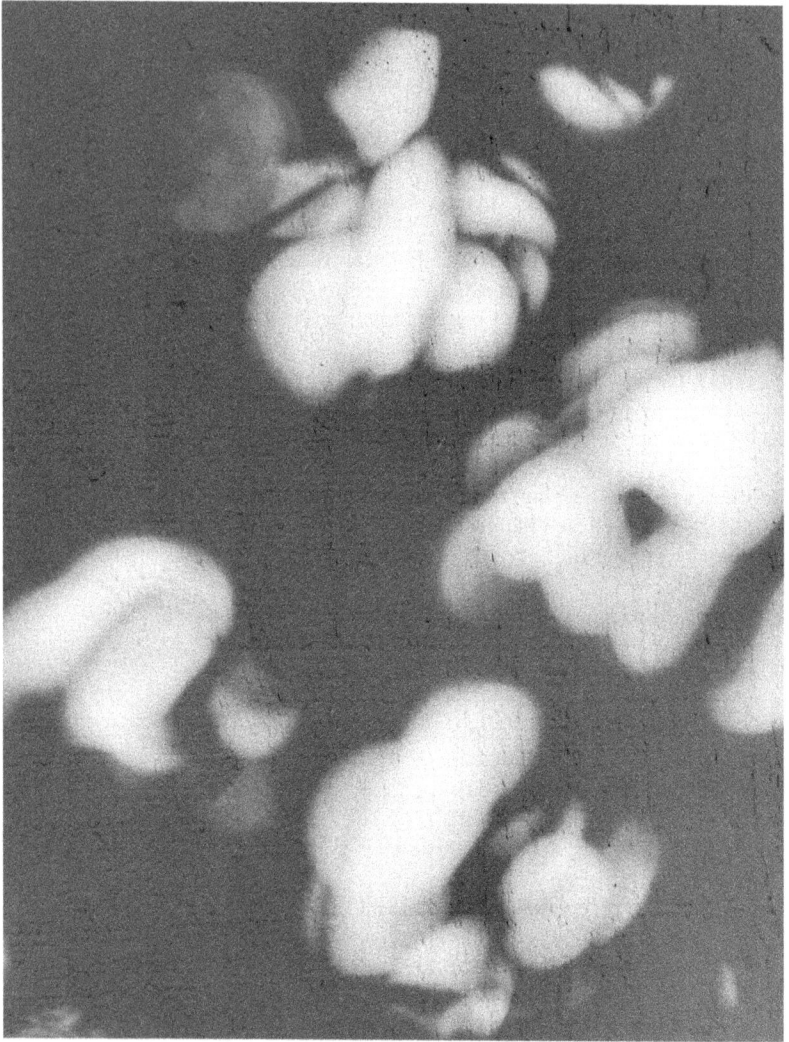

III.

Here's How It Will Go

The chest cage and diaphragm, with expansive spirit,
cooperate one last time,
the discomfort at the depth of the intake
a reason to pause, with a sense of fullness
if not quite fulfillment;
there may be a last perception of aroma
attending the secretive swirling
within those dark cavernous hollows,
and maybe I will still hear
my own last letting go
my sigh in accepting that pain or fear or relief,
that last passive expulsion of vital and toxic gases,
from the elaborate labyrinth on which I've so long depended,
without seeing it, or knowing its real intricacy, hardly even aware of it,
throughout all the hoarse wet wheezing,
and the dry coarse coughing, and
whatever eloquence and beneficence I could muster,
to balance the ugly exclamations to which I duly confess,
the controlled expressions of my limited emotional range, or
the uncontrolled expressions of my limited emotional range,
as if those vocalizations, the manipulations of airy elements,
were some essence of me, and who I was for those moments,
defining some idea of me; of course, yes, I would have that thought,
even as the oxygen, lasting through that final breath,
is conclusively released from its captured exploitation,
allowing that thought, perhaps, to somehow seem to cease.

Death Certificate Instructions

"The cause-of-death information should be YOUR best medical OPINION. A condition can be listed as "probable" even if it has not been definitively diagnosed."
[CDC https://www.cdc.gov/nchs/data/dvs/blue_form.pdf]

You are not to write: "old age," "infant prematurity," "heart stopped," or "wouldn't breathe," "lost the will to live," "recalled by his God" or "became overtly inert to be subsumed by her elemental universe."

You have a responsibility to the accuracy of the statistics, so that each of us count for something, even just a data point that may ultimately represent a person to a future curiosity, which might wonder at the documentation of this death, the text revealing how the form filler was taught to judge it.

There are four lines in Part I. If you can opine, summarize why this person, once living, is no longer living, the ultimately fatal "chain of events." Do so tersely, not mentioning kindness, meanness, bliss or agony, refrain from recounting laughter or tears, the subtlety and nuance of understandings and misunderstandings, but why, in your estimation of linear causality, the person's body is there, while you are filling out this form over here.

The example is instructive: "Line a. Immediate Cause: Rupture of Myocardium; Onset to Death: Minutes." One is not to write "broken heart," even though cardiologists say there are myriad ways that hearts can break. Hearts can be mended, they tell us, not forever; no one says that, and it's not usually explicitly stated that all we have is just temporary.

The other lines are to list sequential underlying causes, listed backwards, so that Line a. is "due to (or a consequence of)" Line b., then Line c., then Line d. Other specialists, now with perfected hindsight, can chime in with their own ideas about such a death, from the geneticist, the pediatrician, the surgeon, the psychiatrist, or pathologist, even though this person's companion or family might really know best. We must acknowledge that the patient or family may choose to not reveal everything, or anything.

There is no fifth line for the necessary antecedent condition of all death, which is birth, certified or not. The death certifiers would rather not think about how religious persons or politicians around the world might conceive the beginning of life differently, or a how to consider a leg just after amputation; realize that a stillbirth requires a completely different form.

Part II. is a blank box for "other significant conditions contributing to death." Probable conditions are allowed, a conventional diagnosis is implied. The example uses diabetes, COPD, and smoking; those persons were a classic stereotype for a certain generation as we form-fillers developed our current mode of etiological thinking.

For probable conditions, one is not to write "free spirit," "innocence," "stubbornness," "willful ignorance," "cowardice," or "heroism." Do not list "living" as a condition, or any joys, distresses, needs or wants, the uncertainties or boredoms in the daily duty of life. Do not note a frameshifted personality, creating that person's uniquely mutated point of view, the antecedents which may have led to the singular sequence to summarize on this form, about a unique life and its irrevocable death.

"IF FEMALE:" has its own box; two of the check box choices are: "Not pregnant, but pregnant within 42 days of death" and "Not pregnant, but pregnant 43 days to 1 year before death."

The certifier knows that women are more than a pregnancy status, but the statisticians evidently have a job to do, this is how they chose to do it, and make us count days here. Perhaps we need explicit instructions, since it must be known that we fail, on our own, to make each day count.

"MANNER OF DEATH" is yet another box to be checked: "Natural / Homicide / Accident / Pending Investigation/ Suicide / Could not be determined" are the options. They do not include "fighting all the way," or "serenely"; the certifier need not be present at the moments when death was imminent, then apparent, or when examined to a certainty.

In Confidence No Longer

for David J. Gale

I wanted to confide in you just now,
even though we hadn't talked in over a year.
I talked then, without much confidence, and you listened,
because you had to, unable to move, the rhythm of your
tracheostomy and ventilator providing a semblance of reply.

The inadequate curtain forced us to pretend our privacy.
Did you think that I poorly masked my private prognosis?
I didn't tell you that I had seen worse, with rare
recoveries, so displaying a muted optimism was genuine.
I wasn't consciously acting; you were better than I'd imagined.

An intern could have predicted your months after that,
with sudden changes, acute transfers, and modern remedies,
but not your unspeaking steelcore resistance to demise.
So when they found you, and said it was a heart attack,
our retreat into disbelief was just as unsurprising.

But I wanted to confide in you just now.
There wasn't much you confided in me, I know;
there was no symmetry, no bartering nor premise
of equity in our sharing; some might have called it fraternal,
familial, or paternal. Maybe an exploitation of friendship.

There was no one else in the rest of the world
in whom I would confide, for so many things.
You accepted the additional burdens with grace.
And I wanted to confide in you just now.

Isolation Cocoon, May 2020

After Zhuangzi's Butterfly Dream

Spinning, what you will, in heeding that swarm of guidance, creating
your own shell, then transforming, as you will, within that isolation,
still seems like an almost unconvincing, almost unnecessary nuisance.

You had chosen this situation, if it is fair to say there was a choice,
when there was no viable alternative. Your cocoon can feel so safe,
an illusion perhaps, but reality provides nothing less vulnerable.

The walls are thin enough to allow you to breathe, and to vaguely hear
or feel vibrations, even though their meaning cannot be known.
Light penetrates, and darkness, too; the changes remain obscure.

Ruminating on that former lifestyle, you can digest time thoroughly,
like those last memorable green leaves of Springtime, then so succulent,
and satisfying, but to what end you know not; not all cocoons survive.

Time, space, being, identity, the interpreted past, the fancied future
can all be consumed within your insatiable capsule; chrysalis or cocoon,
distinctions no longer matter; each benefits from a covering and distancing.

Complacency or contentment allows a concentration on one's only
certainty, the presentness right now, in this cell-like confinement,
because emergence would require several just preposterous miracles.

Emerging from an Isolation Cocoon, 2022

"The caterpillar does all the work but the butterfly gets all the publicity."
~Attributed to George Carlin

The security layers started peeling away, seemingly too soon.
Once constricting, every movement and moment a struggle,
who would guess that the loosening would be so worrying?

Preposterous miracles had manifested themselves, albeit
imperfectly; so one emerges, reviving afresh in the sunlight, imbibing
the unmasked scents, even as the serial-killing fiend remains free.

A *kaleidoscope* of butterflies is what one calls a mass fluttering;
that term could well apply to humans here, self-identifying their
variants and varieties of existence, behaviors, and beliefs.

The excess of losses has been unthinkable, and not to be forgotten.
Preventive interventions were knowingly imprecise, but lacking
protections from denials was also hazardous for the republic's health.

Poets have long lyricized ideal truth, but the pandemic taught
how fragile truth can be, the fragile beauty of a glistening bubble,
buffeted almost to bursting by a cacophony of ravenous twittering.

Yet one can now stretch out shimmering wings, so to speak,
with the brash confidence befitting a monarch, fully expecting
to start a new cycle in life, despite the circling shadows overhead.

**The Professor of Medicine Demonstrates
Conversing with a Patient, Displaying Vocal Nuance
to Impart Subtleties, like Empathy, a Humane
Concern, a Willingness to Be Helpful, along
with Erudition and Experience That Implies a
Practical Wisdom, a Contemporary Respect
and Affirmation for a Person's Uniqueness,
Projecting a Sense of Enveloping Confidence
with Confidentiality, Plus a Tacit
Presentation of Principled Honesty
and Ethical Care, Which Many Will Hear,
Though Few Will Really Understand,
an Interpreter's Dream but a Translator's
Nightmare, with the Clearest Conveyance
of Meaning When Intoned, While
Deliciously, Ingenuously Ambiguous When Written
to Be Read, Although Never Meant to Be Recorded
in the Medical Record**

Uh-huh.

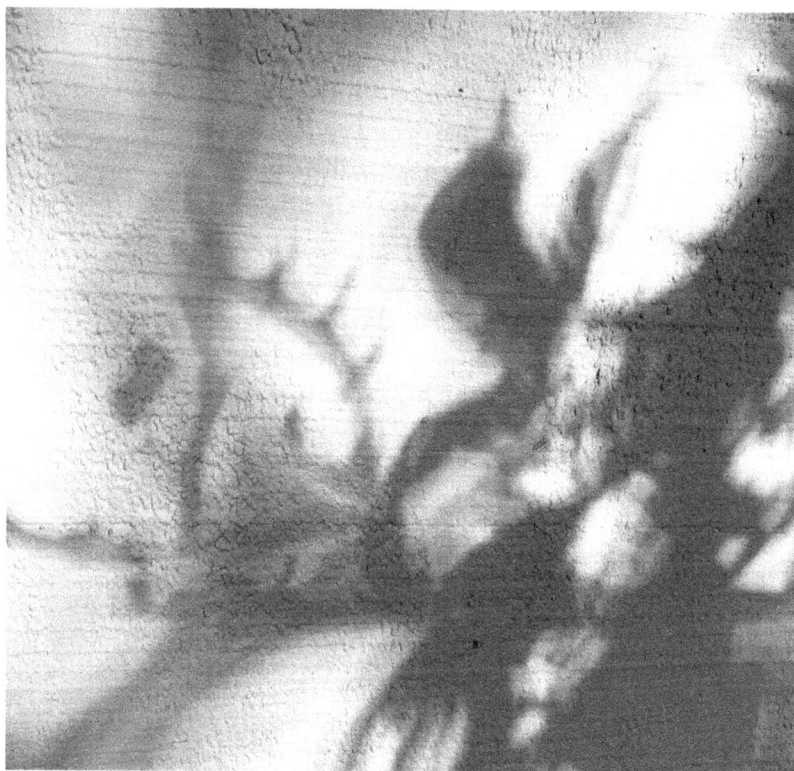

IV.

Hummingbirds, Nosediving

I want to know what it is like for a bat to be a bat. Thomas Nagel

"Hummingbirds,
nosediving…"

Murmured aloud,
vaguely metrical,

while no one is listening,
so hesitantly mumbled.

Aerial displays have a purpose
that the bird surely knows,

be it a flourishing, mate-making
or mortal combat,

a marvelous arc of seeming
elegance, control and precision,

perhaps mundane
to those avian eyes.

It might mean defeat, success,
pleasure, or a just way there.

An optimist, not even bothering
"what it is like" to fly like that,

whose own philosophy leads him
to hear and see lyricism instead,

finds a feathery satisfaction, so what
if he fools himself, again.

Cassiopeia's Dust

Abstract: A dilettante admires a constellation from a hot tub, and considers it the next day. Is it a prose poem, creative nonfiction, or "light" verse, phenomenology, astrophysics, metaphysics or half-lit paronomasia?

A photon hit my retina. Again, again; others also hit. The sensation seemed continuous, albeit twinkling, rather than as discrete and separated points. It was like dust, but I did not blink.

It came from a thing I would call bright, in front of me, over my head, on a dark night; it is said to be a star from the cluster of a pattern I learned to call Cassiopeia, and just in a similar way, I learned about my retina, and I learned about photons, and I learned that some consider them a duality of either wavering or unwavering continuity or perhaps some discretion, meanwhile calling attention to my own uncertainty, and from a source thought to be over 10,000 years away, if one could ever travel at the speed of light, traveling for at least that long, starting before my retina existed to be hit, somehow seeming yellowish to me, when I perceived it, if you made me explain that almost forgotten moment, using the prosaic unmusical vernacular that you are reading as I am using it today. That moment might have been poetic.

Using the word "again" implies a passage of time, but I am not counting. It is as if the photon that hit at least one of my retinal rods, and started the cascade of physico-chemical neuro-electrical events that culminated in my striking down, with my left fourth fingertip, the key for the letter "w" on this keyboard, already the next day, to finish the word now, was aimed for that rod. Perhaps the photon distinguished itself, then extinguished itself, right then, or perhaps, like a visitor in disguise, now seems native, absorbed in my own fabric somehow.

Maybe it was not a single photon or many photons, but another energy some say is also emanating from Cassiopeia, bathing my whole being but evading the notice of my other senses, without an evocative hum or aroma or taste or texture or temperature or pain, motivating my biological machinery from sedation to this creation, although no matter nor energy was created nor destroyed, I do not think, in typing this, but I really have no way of knowing.

This whole conceptual construct might be debatable, if one would bother. The construct fits into my head, if that's where a construct can be found, if findable, and if a construct has dimensions, if measurable, to be fitted, as I am using the word right now. Yes, some demand that reality be measurable and repeatedly so, but as I write, again, I am not counting.

Good science allows me to declare that I am being conditional about it all, and about how I am communicating this way, allowing an exercise of my seldomly used subjunctive voice, as if there were a statistical aspect, perhaps a freedom, if that is how one can characterize a possible lack of pre-determinism, involved in my typing this period.

How you might read this or say this, with what sound or accent of your own, with what connotation or nuanced memory, is of minuscule interest to me, yet here I am typing it for you. If human bodies are made of stardust, or at least contain star photons, from stars like Cassiopeia A, as that remnant might be called, does it follow that this conceptual construct, perhaps labelled a prose poem, perhaps creative nonfiction, is then necessarily stardust, or not necessarily.

A Bird Twitches, Then Disappears

Dull, heavy, and palpable, the single sound
disrupted a reverie. Through the glass,
I saw two birds, grey, white and brown speckled.

One was standing, alert, head cocked and scanning.
I'm not a birdwatcher, but even I could tell
that the one lying on its back appeared unnatural.

It was only the size of my open palm.
As I watched, its intricately spiked right talon
twitched once, then remained still. There was no sound.

Moments passed as I stared. Was there a liquid
at its beak, or around its head? The standing bird
had already flown away, needing to be elsewhere.

I could not recall a bird shriek, or cawing, or
the rustle of a flock or even a single bird's fluttering;
the thudding appearance became an abrupt intrigue.

I looked down at my own open palm, to
gauge its size, to gauge the bird, to
gauge this moment as the bird lay still.

My palm was the perfect size to cradle
the creature, as it seemed to be attaining perfection.
The open hand was also the perfect size

to have swatted that bird down, if it ever
had that intention or inclination, or skill,
in need, or in cruelty, or in jest,

the perfect size to have proffered
a tenderness, a soothing caress; from
cruelty to gentleness, all human intrusions.

As I regarded my palm, its creased and mottled flesh,
the faintest susurration arose, and when I turned,
the bird had vanished, leaving no trace of its being.

The fictions now multiplied:
the quietest predator had swooped in,
carrying away its still warm prey,

or the bird was now resurrected,
perhaps just stunned for that moment,
oblivious to observations and opinions,

the victim of an atmospheric
collision, or concussion, whether
romantic or hostile or accidental.

Or was it that improbable bird, so fallible
as to tumble from the sky, debunking
the dogma of an impeccable Nature,

possibly so senseless with pleasure,
the rising ecstasy for once
quashing its forceful mandate to fly,

choosing to abandon control, aimlessly
allowing fate and wind and gravity
to have their own stochastic ways,

now suddenly compelled to awaken, to rustle itself,
and finding the apparatus unbroken,
restoring breath and the blue sky again soaring;

or was it all the rapture of a reader,
generating an apprehension of grounded things
out of the nebulous thin air of a hushed morning.

Mrs. C.D.B. Stewart, Amongst Writers

Her measured cadence, slow, articulate, and taut-lipped,
swept all of us forward with meticulous craft.

Demarking caesuras with shallow breaths,
she spoke as one might read, with that imperial
and literary accent, the remnant of a once-bright regime.

Echoes of her vanquished brash voicing,
now rasping and plying patrician pleasantries,
enchanted our huddle of aspirants.

"One need not concentrate…," she would intone,
"on discovering the aching secret of life;
rather, focus only upon its gritty details;

for the truest secrets lie therein;
you may look to the balm of that vast ocean, but study
its cresting wave of debris, its intricate teeming debris."

She would pause, with a smile beyond any embarrassment,
or diffidence for homilies, or awkward pretensions of a phrase,
no longer annoyed with a need for uniqueness.

And she insisted upon her pleasure in gin and cigarettes,
even after the chest pains, the wheezes,
the anxious refrains, when her lips then surrendered

their purest azure hues, like the warm effusive waters,
upon which she loved to dwell, aboard the civil yachts,
running free of the shoals in the sun,

erratic, hot rushes of breeze
billowing their spinnakers to sea.

Time Frog Continuum

The ancient pond
A frog leaps in
The sound of the water.
(Matsuo Basho, translated by Donald Keene)

Haiku ancient, here,
now, across geography,
languages and time.

Ageless pond. Then frog,
as destiny compels, jumps,
ceasing the silence.

Frog old, pond ancient,
one panoramic vision
noisily disturbed.

Old frog blinks, but now
listening, longing; lowing,
slow then staccato.

Suddenly silent
a time frog continuum
forever present.

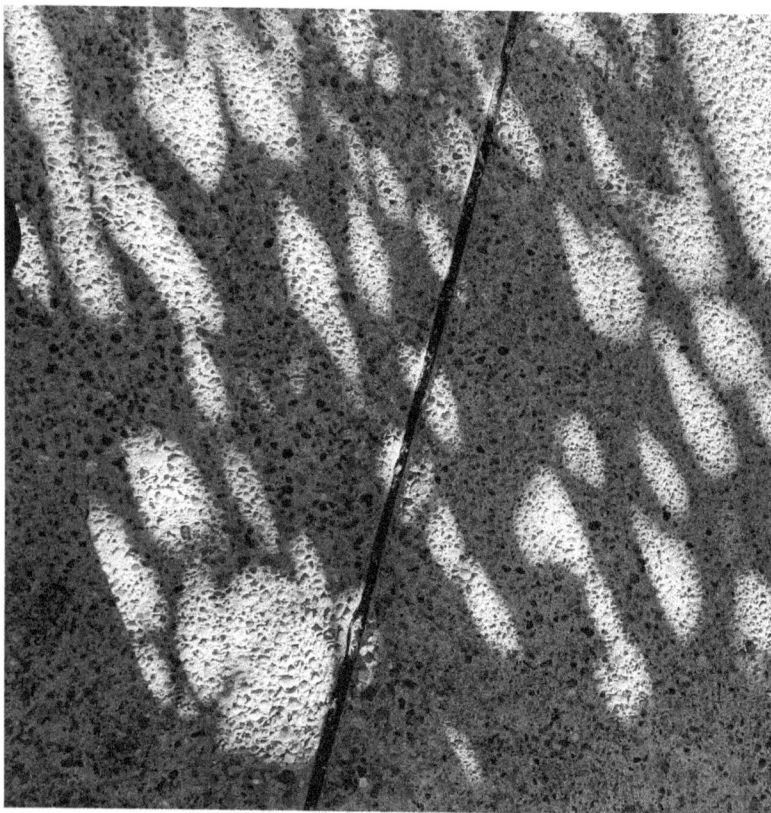

V.

The Ambiguous Life of an Incorrigible Liar

Terrible liar that I am, the twinkle in my eye
that would betray me is really just a cataract.

But I also display an uncontrolled grimace,
which one could equivocally interpret

as winsome, mischievous, or boyish,
rather than as cynical, sly, or ironic.

I am getting away with it again.

My story is a twin volume of fiction,
the mirror images distorting one another.

Terrible Liar and *Terrific Liar* are the titles,
as if the fabric of truth could rip both ways.

Wonderful Liar and *Woeful Liar*, wonky
yet witty, wily yet waggish, will work.

You tell me, what is the difference?

The novelties have been rejected
so many times; unsolicited, but anyway

tossed across those many dim transoms,
into who knows what, or where, without

wondering how or why one would read them.
Most replies or answers are not definitive.

Is here where the duplicity is working, no?

Imagining Sisyphus Happy

"The struggle itself towards the heights is enough to fill a man's heart.
One must imagine Sisyphus happy". *Albert Camus, translated by Justin O'Brien.*

One can not ignore
the boulder, roaring down
again,
its chaotic rumble,
not musical,
lacking color, no setting sun,
but crashing against the sharded
emptiness
no matter how one is inclined.

The completedness
of the quotidian
chore
even after the count is lost,
may just be enough,
if one ignores Sisyphus
himself defining
happiness,
for what one might call a purpose.

Neologician's Grieving Telegramissive

Abysm Betwixt
Coldly Dominates;
Efforts Futilistic,
Gnashingly Harsh
Insensitive Jaggering,
Knackering Lubricious
Memories: Neverevermore.
Oppressively Pirahanical,
Quashing Rebelldemptions,
Scorching Tears,
Uvulating Vulgarity,
Wearyingly Xenocentric;
Zeronisticism.

[added note: sometimes "there are no words;"
here there is no "Y",
no Rhyme nor Reason (mayhap)]

Coiled Twisted

for S.M.

worn rope rough
fibrous razors
ready
to fray further

or flay flesh
not tough enough;
relentless in
exposing underneath

the rawest rubor
the rawest dolor
the rawest calor
the rawest valor

sinuous
resilience
persisting
resisting

Substitutions

The void between us
is now diminishing.
No, that's not right, it was never
infinite or deep. Too dramatic. Chasm?
No. Really no. Chasm isn't right either.

Even when we did touch,
was there that theoretical gap,
a molecular force so strong
that coerced a separation, or
a provocative magnetic repulsion,
now seemingly naive and figurative?
Warping space-time is just too precious.

Your voice is not now at all apparent;
its absolute absence splintering stillness,
a cutting contrast to the clanging
of my own hideous idiocy,
blaring awry, uncontrollably louder.

So many damn devices and platforms,
so many insalubrious sullen insensible
words soiling these pristine pages;
yes, they occupy time and waste time,
each an effort, from one or from many,
awaiting an act of consumption, as if that
would fulfill a pathetic proof of living.

You are now teaching me
that our vocabulary is starkly finite,
that the connotations of synonyms
and antonyms may get closer
to what might be a meaning,
but they don't quite fit, do they;
there is no ready substitute
for not quite fitting. There is not now
nor even then a way to substitute
for how we did fit and didn't quite fit.

Pianist Playing "Blackbird"

Blackbirds do not fly backwards
neither will my mind,
not finding when I must have
first heard the delicate phrasing
that even I can recognize,
young Paul then singing
like the tallest choirboy,
hardly older than me;
how had he known torment,
then create a modulated lightness,
feathering subcutaneous sorrows
with a keystroked heart
careening so close
to the dangerous downdrafts.

Her pirouetting persists,
framing a frottage of fragments
faithfully freeing her fingertips
daring to ascend an acrobatic aerie.

Recurrent Viewing

Is it really the shadowing,
drawing the roundedness
of curves, that allows
sensuality in likeness?

Is it really the shadowing,
missing in the memory
groping for roundedness,
only finding a flattening?

Shadowing our tenuous
perception enhances illusions,
visions, so that the limited light
borders on being adequate.

Shadowing graphite and dust,
peppering the panorama,
diminute in dimensionality,
tower over the ephemera,
and now has to be enough.

For You. You Too.

Hey. You know I did not write this
specifically for you, but you
picked it up anyway. I am not
going to thank you, because your
choices are your own. Many
learn to live with their choices,
not that they have a choice
of unknowable consequences.

Now that you have read this far,
you might be wondering
if this is what you thought it might be,
whether it is really worth any more
of the diminishing time in your life
to read past the next period.

I do not know how you found me
and I do not care to know.
The question of why I wrote this
will not be answered to you,
although it is in a language that you
can presumably read.

Understanding is not my concern.
I do not want to hear your accent
if you read this out loud.
These words are the incentive
to never find me again.

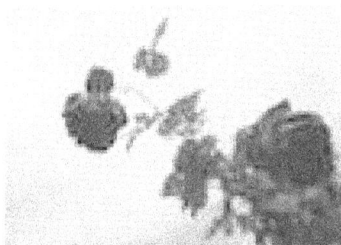
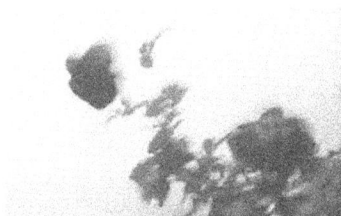
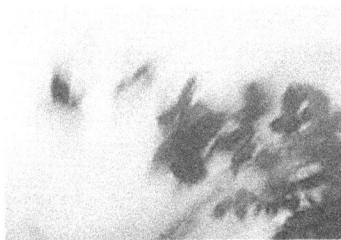

Acknowledgements
(poems previously published, edited here to fit format)

Cassiopeia's Dust. *Philosophy and Literature, Apr 2021.*
https://muse.jhu.edu/pub/1/article/796842

Chief Complaint: He Predicts Earthquakes. *BMJ: Medical Humanities.*
2017;43:e29. https://mh.bmj.com/content/43/3/e29

Couplets to a Pre-Existing Condition. *Pediatrics 1995.*
https://pediatrics.aappublications.org/content/95/3/330

Emerging from an Isolation Cocoon 2022. *CDC Emerging Infectious
Diseases, July 2022.* https://wwwnc.cdc.gov/eid/article/28/7/22-0488 article

Handwashing 03:47. Published with editorial mistakes. *JAMA*
2018;319(24):2561. https://jamanetwork.com/journals/jama/fullarticle/2685991

Here's How It Will Go. *Pangyrus 2020.*
https://www.pangyrus.com/poetry/heres-how-it-will-go/

Isolation Cocoon, May 2020. *CDC Emerging Infectious Diseases, Nov 2020.*
https://wwwnc.cdc.gov/eid/article/26/11/20-2993 article

Matter of Fact. *Neurology® 2018;* 90:139. https://n.neurology.org/content/
neurology/90/3/139.full.pdf. *Audio:* NPub.org/5kr93u

Missing Any Thing. *Maya's Micros ed. 4 / Batch 009 / The Closed Eye Open,
Nov 2020.* https://theclosedeyeopen.com/mayas-micros-ed-4/

Mrs. C.D.B. Stewart, Amongst Writers. *Cathexis NW 2019.*
https://www.cathexisnorthwestpress.com/post/mrs-c-d-b-stewart-amongst-writers

"Neologician's Grieving Telegramissive." in *Remembering Wallace Stevens,*
ed. John Lavin, *Moonstone Arts Center, Phila. PA, 2025, pg.38.*

The Chief Poisoner Will See You Now. *Antiphon. 2019, Issue 24, pg 9-10.*
https://drive.google.com/file/d/1uD-iqQ9hRhWJ4gC9Q3 unNvP-UkwXgsl/view

The Professor of Medicine… *leaflet-ejournal, Permanente Journal, 2020.*
http://www.leaflet-ejournal.org/archives-index/item/professor-of-medicine

Time Frog Continuum, abridged from a haiku cycle:
https://www.origamipoems.com/poets/489-ron-louie

Tonio Telling Time. *BMJ: Medical Humanities*. 2017;43:e34.
https://mh.bmj.com/content/43/3/e34

What the Magician Whispered. *Maya's Micros, ed. 15 /Batch 033 / The Closed Eye Open, March 2022.*
https://theclosedeyeopen.com/mayas-micros-ed-15/

A Bird Twitches, Then Disappears; Counting to Himself, Again; Retrogenesis as Oxymoron; Our Dancing vs. Wrestling Moves all appeared as earlier versions on the https://CareGivingOldGuy.website

Readings available through links:

Audio recording, *The Chief Poisoner*:
https://soundcloud.com/search?q=antiphon louie

Audio recording, *Matter of Fact*:
https://cdn-links.lww.com/permalink/wnl/a/
wnl_90_3_2017_12_08_louie_848168_sdc1.mp3

CDC Podcasts:

Isolation Cocoon, May 2020:
https://tools.cdc.gov/medialibrary/index.aspx#/media/id/482525

Emerging from an Isolation Cocoon, 2022 :
https://tools.cdc.gov/medialibrary/index.aspx#/media/id/730951

Ron Louie has been a pediatric oncologist, dementia primary caregiver, clinical investigator, administrative chief and is now a retired clinical professor. This is a revised collection of his poems, along with new poems. Other writings include medical and non-fiction pieces.

His work as an Alzheimer home caregiver is the subject of blog posts on AlzheimerGadfly.net and CareGivingOldGuy.website.

This chapbook is meant to be easily shared. Lines may be quoted, if the chapbook or original publication source is cited, but it is copyrighted, not to be abused or pirated without permission.

If so moved, the reader could consider a donation to the **Make-A-Wish Foundation**, https://wish.org/akwa or the **Children's Oncology Group Foundation**, https://thecogfoundation.org . Ron has been a donor.

.